WHAT THEY WON'T TELL YOU ABOUT HYPERTENSION: NUTRITIONAL SECRETS FOR HIGH BLOOD PRESSURE

By: Cedric Williams, Concerned Pharmacist

"High blood pressure isn't just a numbers game—true control comes from nourishing your body with the right nutrients, not simply cutting salt. Balance your minerals, heal naturally, and reclaim your health."

Introduction

If you're reading this, you're likely exhausted from trying to make sense of the conflicting advice surrounding blood pressure. You've been told to cut salt, reduce fats, and measure every nutrient you consume—yet the results just don't add up. Despite following all the conventional guidelines and taking the prescribed medications, your blood pressure remains a constant, frustrating battle.

While medications can be effective in managing blood pressure, they often come with potential side effects. For instance, beta-blockers can cause fatigue and depression, while diuretics may lead to dehydration or electrolyte imbalances. Over time, some people experience even more serious health concerns like kidney damage, nutrient depletion, or an increased risk of diabetes. Many patients feel stuck, relying on these drugs while their underlying health issues remain unresolved.

This book is here to provide you with an alternative approach—one that empowers you to address the root causes of high blood pressure through diet, lifestyle changes, and a deeper understanding of your body's natural healing abilities.

I've seen this struggle firsthand, both as a pharmacist and personally, now that I've reached middle age. Like many of you, I'm desperate to find novel ways to stay ahead of Father Time and avoid the decline that so many accept as inevitable. But as I started questioning my own health, I also began rethinking what I had been taught about managing hypertension and overall well-being.

Here's what they don't tell you: the real issue often isn't as simple as cutting salt. In fact, many of the guidelines we follow are heavily influenced by Big Pharma, which prioritizes medication over natural, sustainable solutions. And while hypertensive drugs may have their place, blindly relying on them isn't necessarily the answer. There's a wealth of data and research out there— evidence that suggests a different approach or at least, a supplemental and preventative approach—but it doesn't easily break through the conventional dogma.

What They Won't Tell You About Hypertension is based on that overlooked research. As a holistic pharmacist, I've come to believe that the body's ability to heal itself is far more powerful than we give it credit for. The medications we take today are derived from nature—plants, minerals, herbs—and yet we often ignore the most accessible medicine we have: the food we eat.

This book isn't about cutting out salt or demonizing fats. It's about using the right nutrients—sodium, potassium, magnesium, fat-soluble vitamins—to allow your body to function at its best. You can manage your blood pressure without feeling deprived, and you don't have to rely solely on medication to do so.

As someone who's now in the thick of middle age, I know firsthand the pressures we face to keep our health in check. We want to stay ahead of the inevitable, and we want real, lasting solutions. This book offers those solutions—based on real research and natural approaches to managing hypertension.

However, this is not a substitute for professional medical advice. Always consult with your doctor before making changes to your health regimen, especially if you are currently on medication. The goal here is to give you knowledge that empowers—not replaces—medical care.

Welcome to a new way of thinking about hypertension, one that puts you back in control of your health and gives you the tools to beat growing old on your own terms.

Table of Contents

<u>**OTHER BOOKS BY THE AUTHOR**</u>

Stay tuned for future works, where I'll continue exploring natural health and challenging conventional wisdom on critical health topics.

In my upcoming books, I'll delve deeper into the cutting-edge science that is reshaping our understanding of human health, uncovering the truths that often get overlooked or dismissed. My work will focus on controversial subjects in health—topics where new scientific evidence offers fresh perspectives that challenge old paradigms.

From nutrition to disease prevention, these books will provide you with the tools and insights needed to make informed choices about your well-being. If you enjoyed my book and found it helpful, please share it and leave a five-star review so that others may be enlightened as well.

Follow me to stay updated on my journey as I continue to question, research, and share natural solutions and breakthrough knowledge that could change how we think about health and wellness.

For a more guided approach, consider using the **Hypertension Management Journal**—designed to help you track your daily progress and keep you on the path to success. Plus, check out my curated **list of recommended products** that support effective blood pressure management, featuring highly-rated best sellers from supplements to home monitoring devices on social media @EnjoyableBook.

Cedric.W.writes@gmail.com

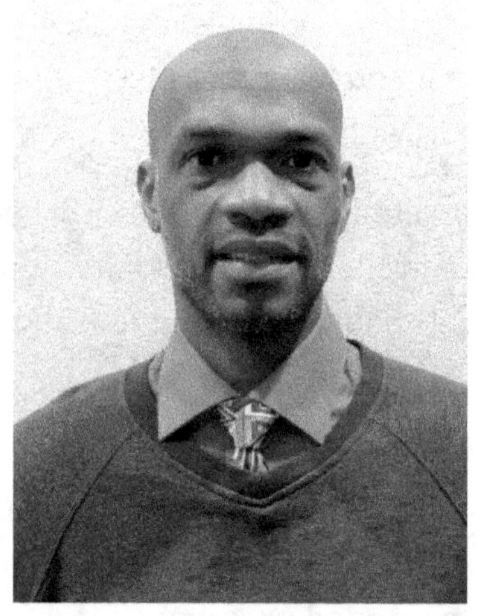

Preface

As I approach almost five decades on this earth, I find myself reflecting on a life deeply intertwined with human biology. For over 30 years, I've been fascinated by how our bodies work—how they respond to what we put in them, what we take away, and how they interact with their environment. The last 21 of those years have been spent focusing on drugs and human biology, and for nearly two decades, I've worked as a licensed pharmacist.

But something changed in me about seven years ago. After years of dispensing medications and watching patients cycle through prescription after prescription, I began to ask myself a different question: What if we could do more to understand, prevent, and even cure chronic diseases rather than just treat the symptoms? What if, instead of reacting to illness, we took steps to ensure our bodies were better equipped to stay healthy in the first place? That's when my journey toward a preventative, natural mindset truly began.

This mindset only grew stronger during the COVID-19 pandemic. The virus was a brutal wake-up call—not just because of its devastating effects on global health but because of the way science, which I had always trusted, became politicized, money-driven, and muddled with power struggles. It seemed to me that amidst the chaos, the essence of true, evolving science—the kind that should grow and adapt as we learn more about the human body—was being drowned out by agendas.

And that's the point: the COVID virus evolves, and science should too, but it's not keeping pace because pharmaceutical companies have a significant influence over what we learn. Our understanding of the human body and disease states should constantly be expanding. That's why I've written this book—not because I have all the answers, but because I want to be part of that evolution. I want to share the new information that's gaining traction, and I want to do it in a way that you can easily understand and apply to your own life and health.

I'm not here to tell you what to think or do. I'm not here to push an agenda. I'm here because, like you, I care about my future health. I care about finding real, sustainable solutions to living well and preventing disease. And after decades of studying the body and its relationship with the medicines we take, I want to share what I've learned, unbiased—and what I'm still learning—so that together, we can move toward a better, more informed future.

This book isn't about quick fixes or following fads. It's about presenting new information in a practical, understandable way. My hope is that by the end, you'll not only feel empowered to take control of your health but also have the tools to make informed decisions that align with your body's natural ability to heal and thrive. Thank you for joining me on this journey.

Chapter 1: Understanding Hypertension: A Symptom, Not a Disease

What is Hypertension?

Hypertension, commonly known as high blood pressure, is a condition that occurs when the force of blood pushing against the walls of your arteries is consistently too high. Blood pressure readings are given in two numbers: systolic (the pressure in your arteries when your heart beats) and diastolic (the pressure when your heart rests between beats). For example, a reading of 120/80 mmHg is considered normal.

However, hypertension isn't a disease in and of itself—it's often a symptom of underlying issues. When you're told you have high blood pressure, it's not just a standalone problem to be managed with medication. It's your body's way of signaling that something else is out of balance, whether it's related to diet, stress, or another health condition. And because hypertension is so often treated as a disease in isolation, the root causes frequently go ignored.

Causes of Hypertension

Primary (Essential) Hypertension

In most cases, hypertension develops with no clear, direct cause—this is called primary or essential hypertension. Several factors can contribute to this form of hypertension, including:

- Genetics: If your parents or close relatives have high blood pressure, you are more likely to develop it.

- Age: As we age, our blood vessels naturally become less flexible, which can lead to increased blood pressure.

- Diet: Diets high in processed foods, salt, and sugar contribute to hypertension by promoting inflammation and nutrient imbalances.

- Lifestyle: Lack of physical activity, obesity, and smoking are significant lifestyle factors that can elevate blood pressure over time.

Secondary Hypertension

Secondary hypertension occurs when high blood pressure is the result of another underlying condition. Unlike primary hypertension, secondary hypertension often has a more specific cause, such as:

- Kidney Disease: When your kidneys aren't filtering fluid properly, it can cause an increase in blood pressure.

- Hormonal Disorders: Conditions such as thyroid imbalances or elevated aldosterone levels (a hormone that regulates salt and water in the body) can contribute to hypertension.

- Sleep Apnea: This condition can cause fluctuations in oxygen levels during sleep, leading to increased blood pressure.

Hypertension, whether primary or secondary, should be viewed as a symptom—your body's way of signaling that something is off. Addressing the root cause is critical for long-term control.

Prevalence of Hypertension

Hypertension is a widespread health issue, affecting millions of people worldwide. According to the CDC and World Health Organization (WHO), approximately 1.13 billion people globally have hypertension. In the United States, nearly half of adults are considered hypertensive under the new guidelines.

- Global Prevalence: Hypertension is more prevalent in low- and middle-income countries, where access to healthcare may be limited. Lifestyle factors such as poor diet and lack of physical activity also contribute to this trend.

- Risk Factors: Individuals over the age of 60, African Americans, and those with a family history of hypertension are at a higher risk of developing high blood pressure. Additionally, lifestyle factors such as stress, excessive alcohol consumption, and poor diet further increase this risk.

Hypertension Diagnosis and Issues with Blood Pressure Monitors

How Hypertension is Diagnosed

Hypertension is generally diagnosed after multiple readings of blood pressure taken over time, either in a clinical setting or at home using a blood pressure monitor. A reading of 130/80 mmHg or higher is now considered hypertension.

Inaccuracies in Diagnosis

Unfortunately, diagnosing hypertension isn't always straightforward. Here are some common issues:

- White Coat Syndrome: Many people experience elevated blood pressure in medical settings due to anxiety, leading to an overdiagnosis of hypertension.

- Masked Hypertension: Conversely, some individuals may have normal blood pressure in a doctor's office but experience elevated readings at home or in daily life, resulting in underdiagnosis.

Issues with Blood Pressure Monitors

Blood pressure monitors are widely used to diagnose and track hypertension, but they have their own set of problems:

- Calibration Problems: Home blood pressure monitors may give inaccurate readings if not properly calibrated. Over time, even high-quality devices can lose accuracy.

- Improper Cuff Size: Using a cuff that is too small or too large for your arm can skew the results. A tight cuff may give a higher reading, while a loose cuff can underreport blood pressure.

- Body Positioning: Incorrect posture while taking your blood pressure—such as crossing your legs or not supporting your arm at heart level—can lead to inaccurate readings.

- Wrist Monitors: While convenient, wrist monitors are generally less accurate than upper-arm monitors because of the narrower blood vessels in the wrist and more variability in positioning.

Over-Diagnosis and Over-Medication

The updated CDC and AHA guidelines that lowered the threshold for hypertension to 130/80 mmHg have led to more people being diagnosed and treated with medication. However, some argue that this can lead to over-medication, especially in individuals whose readings are only slightly elevated or fluctuate due to temporary stress or environmental factors. Many of these individuals may not require aggressive treatment.

Common Classes of Medications for Hypertension

While medication is often prescribed to manage hypertension, it's important to understand how these drugs work and the potential side effects associated with each:

- ACE Inhibitors: These medications help relax blood vessels by preventing the formation of a chemical that tightens them. Common side effects include a persistent cough and elevated potassium levels.

- Beta-Blockers: These reduce heart rate and the force of the heart's contractions. Side effects may include fatigue, cold hands, and possible depression.

- Diuretics: Often called "water pills," these medications help eliminate excess salt and water through urination. However, they can cause dehydration, electrolyte imbalances, and kidney issues if used long-term.

- Calcium Channel Blockers: These prevent calcium from entering cells of the heart and blood vessel walls, relaxing blood vessels.

Side effects can include dizziness, swelling, and constipation.

- ARBs (Angiotensin II Receptor Blockers): Similar to ACE inhibitors, ARBs prevent blood vessels from tightening but with fewer side effects. They are a preferred alternative for patients who cannot tolerate ACE inhibitors.

While these medications can lower blood pressure, they often come with side effects, including long-term risks such as nutrient depletion (magnesium, potassium), kidney damage, or the development of type 2 diabetes.

Concerns with CDC Blood Pressure Guidelines

In 2017, the CDC and AHA lowered the threshold for hypertension diagnosis from 140/90 mmHg to 130/80 mmHg. This change dramatically increased the number of people classified as hypertensive, especially among older adults. However, there are concerns that this shift may lead to over-medication, particularly in individuals who may not need such aggressive treatment.

Why This Could Be Dangerous

Emerging research suggests that aggressively lowering blood pressure to less than 130/80 mmHg may actually increase mortality in certain populations, particularly frail older adults. According to a study focusing on blood pressure management in individuals over 75, those with systolic blood pressure below 130 mmHg showed a higher risk of mortality compared to those maintaining blood pressure in the 140-160 mmHg range. For individuals over 85, this risk becomes even more pronounced.

This evidence challenges the one-size-fits-all approach of current guidelines, emphasizing that for some individuals, especially the elderly, aiming for such low blood pressure targets may do more harm than good. The study concludes that particularly in frail older adults, blood pressure management should be more individualized, taking into account overall health and other co-existing conditions rather than strictly focusing on achieving a target below 130/80 mmHg.

By treating hypertension as a symptom of underlying health conditions and not merely a standalone disease, healthcare providers can adopt a more cautious, patient-centered approach to blood pressure management—one that may ultimately reduce unnecessary medication and potential harm.

What's New About Hypertension: Insights from Recent Research

Emerging research continues to reshape how we understand hypertension:

- Hypertension as a Symptom: Hypertension is often a sign of underlying metabolic imbalances, chronic stress, or inflammation. By treating the root causes, we may be able to reduce or eliminate hypertension naturally.

- Role of Nutrients: Nutritional imbalances—especially in potassium, magnesium, and calcium—are increasingly recognized as key factors in managing blood pressure.

- Impact of Gut Health: Gut health plays a larger role in blood pressure than previously thought. Endotoxins produced by gut bacteria can contribute to inflammation, which in turn affects blood pressure regulation.

- Cellular Energy Imbalance: Recent studies suggest that poor cellular energy production is linked to hypertension, emphasizing the need to address overall metabolic health.

- Beyond Sodium: While sodium intake has long been a focus, newer studies suggest that balancing sodium with potassium and magnesium is more effective in managing blood pressure than simply reducing sodium.

A New Perspective on Hypertension

Hypertension is a symptom of deeper issues within the body, and it should be treated as such. By addressing the root causes—whether through diet, stress management, or natural supplementation—you can reduce your reliance on medications and take control of your long-term health. Understanding the bigger picture will empower you to make informed decisions about your treatment and work toward lasting wellness.

Chapter 2: The Salt Myth Uncovered

For decades, we've been told to fear salt. Doctors, nutritionists, and health guidelines have warned us to limit our sodium intake, claiming it's a leading cause of high blood pressure and heart disease. Supermarkets are filled with "low-sodium" products, and restaurant menus often boast dishes that minimize salt. But what if we've been led astray? What if the real story behind salt and hypertension is far more nuanced—and less alarming—than we've been taught?

This chapter is about unraveling the confusion, starting with the history behind the "low-salt" movement and diving into the science that challenges this long-standing belief. We'll take a close look at what recent research says about sodium, the body's actual needs, and how salt interacts with other key minerals like potassium, magnesium, and calcium to maintain proper health. The truth is, salt isn't the villain it's been made out to be— and cutting it from your diet may not be the answer to lowering your blood pressure.

The History Behind the "Low-Salt" Advice

The story begins in the mid-20th century when scientists first began to investigate the link between salt intake and high blood pressure. One of the earliest studies that fueled the low-salt narrative was conducted on patients with hypertension who showed a reduction in blood pressure when their salt intake was drastically reduced. These findings quickly led to the belief that less salt equals healthier blood pressure.

However, there was one major flaw with these early studies: they focused on extreme cases of hypertension and didn't consider the full picture of human nutrition or the importance of sodium balance. What started as a well-meaning recommendation for a specific group of people soon morphed into a blanket rule for the entire population, and the fear of salt took root in public health guidelines.

Why Sodium is Essential for Health

The truth is that sodium is not the enemy. In fact, it's essential for many critical functions in the body. Sodium plays a major role in maintaining fluid balance, nerve function, and muscle contraction. Without enough sodium, your body struggles to regulate these processes, which can lead to dehydration, fatigue, and even dangerous electrolyte imbalances.

The body needs a certain amount of sodium to maintain homeostasis—a state of balance where everything from blood pressure to muscle function operates smoothly. When sodium levels drop too low, the body compensates by releasing hormones that increase blood pressure, creating the exact problem that we're trying to avoid. In other words, the very advice to cut salt may be leading to the high blood pressure it's trying to prevent.

The Difference Between Processed Salts and Natural Sea Salt

Not all salts are created equal. Much of the confusion around sodium and hypertension stems from the type of salt we're consuming. Highly processed table salt, stripped of its natural minerals and often laden with additives like anti-caking agents, behaves differently in the body than natural sources of salt, like sea salt or Himalayan salt.

Natural sea salts are rich in trace minerals like magnesium, potassium, and calcium, which help balance sodium levels and support cardiovascular health. These trace minerals are often missing in processed table salt, making it harder for your body to maintain the proper electrolyte balance needed for optimal blood pressure. By choosing more natural sources of salt, you're not just adding flavor to your food—you're nourishing your body with the minerals it needs to keep blood pressure in check.

The Truth about how Salt Intake Affects Blood Pressure when Balanced with Other Minerals

The relationship between salt and blood pressure isn't as simple as "more salt equals higher blood pressure." It's about balance. Sodium works in tandem with other minerals—especially potassium, magnesium, and calcium—to regulate blood pressure. When these minerals are out of balance, your body struggles to maintain proper blood pressure levels.

For instance, potassium helps to counteract the effects of sodium by relaxing blood vessels and aiding in the elimination of excess sodium through urine. Magnesium and calcium also play critical roles in regulating muscle contraction and fluid balance. When you have adequate levels of these minerals, your body can handle a higher sodium intake without raising your blood pressure. The problem arises when modern diets—low in whole foods and rich in processed options—are deficient in these minerals, leading to an imbalance.

Recent studies suggest that the key to managing blood pressure isn't necessarily reducing salt but rather ensuring you get enough of these other minerals. By consuming a diet rich in potassium, magnesium, and calcium—through foods like leafy greens, fruits, nuts, and dairy products—you can help your body maintain a healthy sodium balance and support cardiovascular health without feeling deprived.

The Takeaway: Embrace Salt in Balance

You don't need to fear salt. It's time to put the myth to rest and take a more balanced approach to sodium in your diet. The key isn't eliminating salt altogether but consuming it wisely, in combination with the right foods that provide the other essential minerals your body needs to regulate blood pressure naturally.

By choosing natural sea salt over processed table salt and incorporating more potassium, magnesium, and calcium into your meals, you can help maintain healthy blood pressure levels without feeling restricted. Embrace salt for what it truly is—a necessary and beneficial part of your health journey, when consumed in balance with other key nutrients. This shift in perspective could be the breakthrough you've been looking for in your battle with hypertension.

In the next chapter, we'll explore the crucial role that potassium, magnesium, and calcium play in managing blood pressure, and how restoring balance among these minerals can lead to lasting cardiovascular health.

Chapter 3: The Power of Potassium, Magnesium, and Calcium

When we think about managing high blood pressure, the conversation almost always revolves around cutting sodium. But that's only one side of the story. What's often overlooked in mainstream health advice is the role of three crucial minerals—potassium, magnesium, and calcium—that work hand-in-hand with sodium to regulate blood pressure and support cardiovascular health. These minerals play a starring role in the delicate balance that keeps your heart and blood vessels functioning properly.

This chapter will uncover why these three minerals are essential for anyone looking to manage hypertension naturally, and how an imbalance can often be the root cause of high blood pressure. When we neglect potassium, magnesium, and calcium, we disrupt the body's natural ability to maintain equilibrium—and that's where the real danger lies.

Balancing Sodium: The Role of Potassium, Magnesium, and Calcium

You've probably heard that potassium helps balance sodium in the body, but what does that really mean? Potassium acts as a counterbalance to sodium, helping to relax blood vessels and ease the pressure that sodium might otherwise exert. When there's too much sodium and not enough potassium, blood vessels constrict, making it harder for the heart to pump blood efficiently. This leads to higher blood pressure, and over time, can contribute to serious cardiovascular issues.

But it doesn't stop with potassium. Magnesium plays a key role in helping blood vessels relax, which further alleviates the pressure on the cardiovascular system. Magnesium also supports the function of potassium and sodium pumps, which are critical for maintaining proper fluid balance and keeping blood pressure in check.

Calcium, often known for its role in bone health, is equally important for heart function. It aids in the contraction and relaxation of blood vessels and helps to maintain proper muscle function, including the muscle of the heart. When calcium levels are too low, blood vessels can constrict, contributing to elevated blood pressure.

Together, these three minerals create a powerful system that balances sodium and ensures that the body's natural rhythms are maintained. When all four (sodium, potassium, magnesium, and calcium) are in harmony, blood pressure is much easier to regulate. The problem is, many people are deficient in one or more of these minerals—often without realizing it.

Signs of Deficiency and How They Contribute to Hypertension

Unfortunately, modern diets—high in processed foods and low in whole, nutrient-dense options—are often lacking in potassium, magnesium, and calcium. When these minerals are missing from the diet, the body struggles to maintain the delicate balance needed for heart health.

Here are some common signs of deficiency for each mineral:

- Potassium Deficiency: If you're not getting enough potassium, you may experience symptoms like muscle cramps, fatigue, and irregular heartbeats. Low potassium levels can also lead to fluid retention, which can increase blood pressure. Over time, insufficient potassium can put added strain on the heart and blood vessels, making hypertension worse.

- Magnesium Deficiency: Magnesium is involved in hundreds of biochemical reactions in the body, so when levels are low, the effects can be widespread. Common signs of magnesium deficiency include muscle twitches or cramps, mood swings, fatigue, and even abnormal heart rhythms. In relation to blood pressure, low magnesium levels can lead to the stiffening of arteries, making it harder for blood to flow freely, contributing to hypertension.

- Calcium Deficiency: While calcium deficiency is often associated with brittle bones, it can also have serious effects on heart health. Without enough calcium, the blood vessels may become overly constricted, leading to increased blood pressure. Signs of calcium deficiency include muscle cramps, brittle nails, and numbness or tingling in the fingers.

Recognizing the signs of deficiency can be the first step in restoring balance and taking control of your blood pressure.

The Best Food Sources of Potassium, Magnesium, and Calcium

The good news is, it's easy to start replenishing these minerals with whole foods. Here are some of the best food sources for each:

- Potassium: Bananas are often the first food that comes to mind when thinking about potassium, but there are many other great sources. Leafy greens like spinach and Swiss chard, sweet potatoes, avocados, and white beans are all rich in potassium. Incorporating these into your meals can help balance sodium levels and improve blood pressure.

- Magnesium: Nuts and seeds, especially almonds, pumpkin seeds, and sunflower seeds, are great sources of magnesium. Dark leafy greens, like kale and spinach, are also excellent. For those who enjoy seafood, fish like mackerel and salmon are high in magnesium, as are whole grains like quinoa and brown rice.

- Calcium: Dairy products, such as milk, yogurt, and cheese, are well-known sources of calcium, but they're not the only options. Non-dairy sources include leafy greens like kale and collard greens, tofu, almonds, and fortified plant-based milks. These foods will provide the calcium you need to support both your bones and cardiovascular health.

Practical Strategies for Incorporating These Nutrients into Your Daily Meals

Now that we know where to find these minerals, how do we ensure we're getting enough? Here are a few practical ways to start integrating more potassium, magnesium, and calcium into your diet without feeling overwhelmed:

1. Add Leafy Greens: Start with a simple change—add a serving of leafy greens to at least one meal each day. Preferably cooked. Whether it's sautéed spinach with your morning eggs or a salad with lunch, this small habit can dramatically increase your

intake of potassium, magnesium, and calcium.

2. Snack on Nuts and Seeds: Keep a handful of almonds, pumpkin seeds, or sunflower seeds on hand for snacking. These are quick, easy sources of magnesium and calcium, and they're also great for heart health in general.

3. Prioritize Whole Foods: When planning meals, aim for whole foods over processed options. Foods like sweet potatoes, avocados, fish, and legumes should be staples in your diet. These will provide the mineral balance you need to keep your heart and blood vessels functioning optimally.

4. Consider a Supplement (if needed): While food should always be the first source of nutrients, some people may need supplements to reach adequate levels of

potassium, magnesium, or calcium—especially if dietary intake is low or deficiencies have been diagnosed. Be sure to consult with your healthcare provider before starting any supplements to ensure they're right for you.

Meats can be a good source of potassium, magnesium, and calcium—but they may not be as rich in these minerals as plant-based sources or dairy. However, they do provide valuable amounts that can contribute to overall mineral balance. Here's a breakdown of how meats provide these minerals:

1. **Potassium**:
    - Meats like chicken, beef, and pork contain moderate amounts of potassium, though they are not as potassium-dense as plant-based sources like leafy greens or avocados. Still, they can

contribute to your daily intake, especially when combined with other potassium-rich foods.

2. **Magnesium**:

   o Meat typically has lower magnesium content compared to nuts, seeds, or dark leafy greens. However, certain types of meat, particularly fish such as salmon and mackerel, are better sources of magnesium. Red meat and poultry contain smaller amounts but still contribute to your magnesium intake.

3. **Calcium**:

   o Meats are not particularly high in calcium, but bones, such as those found in canned fish like sardines and salmon (when eaten with the bones), are a good source of calcium. Traditional meats like chicken, beef, and pork generally don't provide much calcium, so it's important to look to dairy or plant-based sources if you need to increase calcium intake.

While meats do provide some of these minerals, they are often better paired with a variety of other foods—such as leafy greens, nuts, seeds, and dairy—to ensure a well-rounded intake of potassium, magnesium, and calcium for heart health and blood pressure management.

Reader Takeaway: Restoring Mineral Balance for Hypertension Control

Balancing minerals is key to managing blood pressure naturally. By understanding how potassium, magnesium, and calcium work together with sodium, and by recognizing the signs of deficiency, you can take control of your cardiovascular health. Start by incorporating more whole foods into your diet that are rich in these essential minerals. Small, manageable changes can make a big difference in restoring equilibrium and reducing hypertension—without feeling deprived.

In the next chapter, we'll dive into the world of fat-soluble vitamins A, D, E, and K—and how they're often the unsung heroes when it comes to maintaining a healthy heart and blood pressure.

Chapter 4: Fat-Soluble Vitamins: A, D, E, K – The Unsung Heroes of Heart Health

When we think about heart health and managing hypertension, fat-soluble vitamins are often an afterthought—if they're thought of at all. Yet, vitamins A, D, E, and K play critical roles in maintaining cardiovascular health and regulating blood pressure. The body stores these vitamins in fatty tissues and the liver, making them available when needed. But they don't just work on their own—they interact synergistically with healthy fats like omega-3s and saturated fats, boosting their benefits for your heart and blood vessels.

In this chapter, we'll explore how these fat-soluble vitamins work to protect against hypertension, how to ensure you're getting enough of them through food, and why you shouldn't fear fats when it comes to supporting your heart.

The Role of Fat-Soluble Vitamins in Hypertension Management

Fat-soluble vitamins are vital for cardiovascular health because they regulate inflammation, support cell growth and repair, and maintain the elasticity of blood vessels. When your body has adequate levels of these vitamins, your heart and blood vessels can function efficiently, helping to prevent the arterial stiffness and inflammation that contribute to high blood pressure.

- Vitamin A: Known for its role in vision and immune health, vitamin A also supports the integrity of blood vessel walls. It helps prevent the oxidative stress that can damage arteries, which is especially important in maintaining the flexibility and function of blood vessels under pressure.

  - Vitamin D: One of the most researched vitamins in relation to cardiovascular health, vitamin D helps regulate blood pressure by controlling calcium levels and preventing the calcification of arteries. Deficiency in vitamin D has been strongly linked to hypertension and an increased risk of cardiovascular disease.

- Vitamin E: A powerful antioxidant, vitamin E protects the heart by reducing oxidative stress and inflammation, both of which are major contributors to high blood pressure. It also helps prevent the oxidation of LDL cholesterol, which can clog arteries and lead to hypertension.

- Vitamin K: Perhaps the most underrated of the fat-soluble vitamins, vitamin K plays a key role in blood clotting and regulating calcium in the bloodstream. Without enough vitamin K, calcium can deposit in the arteries rather than in the bones, leading to stiffening of the blood vessels and an increase in blood pressure. Vitamin K2, in particular, has been shown to reduce arterial calcification, supporting heart health.

The Synergistic Effect of These Vitamins with Healthy Fats

Fat-soluble vitamins rely on dietary fat for proper absorption and utilization in the body. This is where the synergy between these vitamins and good fats—such as omega-3s and saturated fats—comes into play. These fats not only help absorb vitamins A, D, E, and K but also work with them to support cardiovascular health.

- Omega-3 fatty acids, found in fatty fish like salmon and mackerel, are known for their anti-inflammatory properties. When combined with vitamin E, they create a powerful defense against oxidative stress, protecting blood vessels from the damage that leads to hypertension.

- Saturated fats, often demonized in mainstream nutrition, are necessary for the absorption of vitamins A, D, E, and K. Sources like butter, coconut oil, and full-fat dairy provide a stable foundation for these vitamins to be absorbed and used effectively by the body. Saturated fats also play a role in cell membrane integrity, which is essential for maintaining the function of cells lining your blood vessels.

By ensuring a balance of these healthy fats in your diet, you can maximize the benefits of fat-soluble vitamins and protect your cardiovascular system.

Practical Ways to Get These Vitamins from Food

Ensuring you get enough of these fat-soluble vitamins doesn't require complicated dietary changes. In fact, many nutrient-dense, whole foods provide an excellent source of these vitamins, along with the healthy fats needed for absorption. Here are some practical ways to incorporate them into your daily meals:

- Vitamin A:

  - Liver (beef, chicken, cod) is one of the richest sources of vitamin A, and even small amounts can provide a significant boost. Eggs and full-fat dairy (butter, cheese) are also great options.

  - Plant-based sources like sweet potatoes, carrots, and spinach provide beta-carotene, a precursor to vitamin A, though it requires fat for conversion.

- Vitamin D:

   - Fatty fish like salmon, mackerel, and sardines are some of the best sources of vitamin D. Egg yolks and fortified dairy products also contribute to your daily intake.

   - While sunlight exposure is a primary source of vitamin D, ensuring you consume these foods can help maintain adequate levels, especially in colder months or for those with limited sun exposure.

- Vitamin E:

   - Nuts and seeds, particularly almonds, sunflower seeds, and hazelnuts, are rich in vitamin E. Avocados and leafy greens like spinach also provide a healthy dose of this antioxidant.

   - Pairing these foods with fats like olive oil or butter can further enhance absorption.

- Vitamin K:

   - Fermented foods, such as natto (a traditional Japanese dish made from fermented soybeans), are rich in vitamin K2, while leafy greens like kale, spinach, and broccoli provide ample amounts of vitamin K1.

   - Animal products, including egg yolks and cheese, are excellent sources of K2, which is critical for preventing arterial calcification.

By focusing on whole, nutrient-dense foods, you can ensure you're getting a balance of these vitamins while supporting your heart health and blood pressure regulation.

How to Avoid Harmful PUFAs While Maintaining Good Fats

While it's important to consume healthy fats for the absorption of fat-soluble vitamins, it's equally important to avoid harmful polyunsaturated fats (PUFAs), which are often found in processed vegetable oils like soybean, corn, and canola oil. These fats can promote inflammation and oxidative stress, contributing to high blood pressure and cardiovascular disease.

Instead, focus on incorporating the following sources of healthy fats:

- Saturated Fats: Found in butter, coconut oil, and full-fat dairy. These fats support cardiovascular health and are stable, meaning they don't oxidize as easily as PUFAs.

- Monounsaturated Fats: Found in olive oil, avocados, and nuts. These fats are heart-healthy and provide a great source of energy while supporting fat-soluble vitamin absorption.

- Omega-3 Fats: Found in fatty fish, flaxseeds, and walnuts. Omega-3s help reduce inflammation and protect against hypertension.

By avoiding processed vegetable oils and focusing on these healthy fats, you can further support your cardiovascular health and enhance the benefits of fat-soluble vitamins.

Reader Takeaway: Harness the Power of Fat-Soluble Vitamins

Fat-soluble vitamins A, D, E, and K are often overlooked in the conversation about heart health, but they play an essential role in managing hypertension and protecting your cardiovascular system. By incorporating foods rich in these vitamins—paired with healthy fats—you can harness their power to support vascular health, reduce inflammation, and maintain balanced blood pressure.

In the next chapter, we'll take a closer look at the role of fats in managing hypertension, particularly debunking the myths around cholesterol and exploring which fats you should embrace for optimal heart health.

Chapter 5: Debunking Dietary Fads: The Truth About Fats and Hypertension

For years, fats have been vilified, especially when it comes to heart health. "Low-fat" has become a buzzword, and many people have been led to believe that reducing fat intake is the key to controlling hypertension and protecting the heart. But what if that advice has been steering us wrong? Recent research has revealed that not all fats are harmful—some are not only beneficial but essential for maintaining a healthy heart and balanced blood pressure.

In this chapter, we're going to break down the confusion surrounding fats, cholesterol, and hypertension. You'll discover why low-fat diets may actually be causing more harm than good, and which fats you should embrace to help regulate blood pressure and support overall cardiovascular health.

Why Low-Fat Diets May Be Doing More Harm Than Good

The rise of low-fat diets can be traced back to the 1960s and 70s, when fat—especially saturated fat—was blamed for the surge in heart disease. Influential studies suggested that dietary fat, particularly from animal sources, was responsible for high cholesterol levels, clogged arteries, and heart attacks. In response, the food industry launched a wave of low-fat products, replacing fat with sugar and refined carbohydrates to keep food palatable.

What followed, however, was not a reduction in heart disease or hypertension but rather an increase in obesity, diabetes, and metabolic disorders—all of which are linked to poor cardiovascular health. As it turns out, removing fat from the diet often leads to overeating refined carbohydrates, which causes spikes in blood sugar and insulin levels, contributing to weight gain and inflammation—two major drivers of high blood pressure.

In reality, fats, particularly the right kinds of fats, are crucial for heart health. They play a role in maintaining cell membrane integrity, producing hormones, and regulating inflammation. Cutting fat out of the diet can disrupt these processes, making it harder to control blood pressure and protect against heart disease.

The Dangers of Processed Vegetable Oils and Trans Fats

While not all fats are bad, certain fats should indeed be avoided—particularly processed vegetable oils and trans fats, which are often found in processed and packaged foods. These harmful fats are highly unstable and prone to oxidation, leading to inflammation and damage to blood vessels.

- Processed Vegetable Oils: Oils like soybean, corn, canola, and sunflower oil are often labeled as "heart-healthy" due to their low levels of saturated fat. However, these oils are rich in omega-6 polyunsaturated fatty acids (PUFAs), which are highly susceptible to oxidation. When these oils oxidize, they generate free radicals that damage cells and blood vessels, leading to inflammation—a major contributor to hypertension. High levels of omega-6 PUFAs, particularly when out of balance with omega-3 fatty acids, have been linked to increased risk of heart disease and high blood pressure.

- Trans Fats: Found in many processed foods and baked goods, trans fats are created by hydrogenating vegetable oils to make them solid at room temperature. These fats are extremely harmful and have been shown to raise LDL (bad) cholesterol, lower HDL (good) cholesterol, and promote inflammation, all of which contribute to hypertension and cardiovascular disease. Fortunately, trans fats are being phased out in many countries, but they can still be found in certain processed products, so it's important to check labels.

By avoiding these harmful fats, you can protect your blood vessels from damage and inflammation and take a major step toward reducing your risk of hypertension.

Healthy Fats for Optimal Blood Pressure Regulation

Now that we've covered which fats to avoid, let's talk about the fats you should be embracing—those that support heart health, reduce inflammation, and help regulate blood pressure.

- Saturated Fats: Contrary to popular belief, saturated fats, found in foods like butter, coconut oil, and full-fat dairy, are not the villains they've been made out to be. These fats are stable and resistant to oxidation, meaning they don't cause the same inflammatory damage as processed vegetable oils. In fact, saturated fats are essential for the proper function of cell membranes and the production of hormones. Studies have shown that including moderate amounts of saturated fats in the diet can actually help regulate blood pressure and improve overall heart health.

- Omega-3 Fats: Found in fatty fish like salmon, mackerel, and sardines, as well as in flaxseeds and walnuts, omega-3 fatty acids are renowned for their anti-inflammatory properties. These fats help to counterbalance the effects of omega-6 fats and reduce inflammation in the blood vessels, which can lower blood pressure. Omega-3s also help improve heart function and protect against arrhythmias and other cardiovascular issues.

- Monounsaturated Fats: Found in foods like olive oil, avocados, and nuts, monounsaturated fats are heart-healthy and can help reduce levels of LDL cholesterol while increasing HDL cholesterol. These fats are also stable and less prone to oxidation, making them a great addition to a diet focused on blood pressure management.

Including these fats in your diet can help you maintain healthy blood pressure, reduce inflammation, and support overall cardiovascular health.

Practical Meal Planning to Include Heart-Healthy Fats

Incorporating healthy fats into your diet doesn't have to be complicated. Here are some practical strategies to ensure you're getting the right fats while avoiding the harmful ones:

1. Cook with Stable Fats: Use saturated fats like butter, ghee, and coconut oil for cooking at higher temperatures. These fats are stable and won't oxidize easily. For lower-temperature cooking or drizzling over salads, opt for heart-healthy olive oil.

2. Include Fatty Fish: Aim to eat fatty fish like salmon, mackerel, or sardines at least twice a week to boost your intake of omega-3 fatty acids. If you're not a fan of fish, consider incorporating flaxseeds, chia seeds, or walnuts into your diet as plant-based sources of omega-3s.

3. Snack on Nuts and Avocados: Monounsaturated fats found in nuts, seeds, and avocados are easy to include in your daily routine. Add a handful of almonds or walnuts to your snacks or slice an avocado onto your salad for a dose of heart-healthy fat.

4. Choose Full-Fat Dairy: Don't be afraid to enjoy full-fat dairy products like cheese, yogurt, and butter. These foods provide saturated fats that support cardiovascular health when consumed in moderation, and they're more satisfying, which can help you avoid overeating.

5. Avoid Processed and Packaged Foods: Processed foods are often loaded with harmful trans fats and oxidized vegetable oils. Stick to whole, unprocessed foods whenever possible, and check labels for hidden sources of unhealthy fats.

Reader Takeaway: Embrace the Right Fats for Heart Health

Not all fats are created equal. While processed vegetable oils and trans fats should be avoided, healthy fats like saturated fats, omega-3s, and monounsaturated fats are essential for heart health and blood pressure regulation. By including these fats in your diet—and ditching the low-fat mindset—you can protect your heart, reduce inflammation, and maintain balanced blood pressure.

In the next chapter, we'll look at how to create a sustainable eating plan that incorporates these heart-healthy fats and minerals, helping you control your blood pressure naturally without feeling restricted or deprived.

Chapter 6: Sustainable Eating for Long-Term Blood Pressure Control

By now, you've learned the importance of balancing minerals, embracing healthy fats, and incorporating fat-soluble vitamins into your diet to manage your blood pressure naturally. But how do you take this information and make it part of your daily life? The key is sustainability—finding an eating plan that nourishes your body without feeling like a burden or leading to deprivation. Restrictive diets are difficult to maintain long-term and often lead to frustration, yet sustainable eating can become second nature.

In this chapter, we'll explore practical ways to create a balanced, nutrient-rich eating plan that supports your cardiovascular health without relying on fads or temporary fixes. You'll find strategies that fit seamlessly into your daily routine, offering lasting benefits for your blood pressure and overall well-being.

Strategies to Create Sustainable, Nutrient-Rich Meals Without Constant Dieting

The first step to sustainable eating is to move away from the idea of "dieting" and instead focus on nourishing your body with foods that support health. Rather than following strict rules or counting calories, aim for balance in every meal. This means including a variety of whole, nutrient-dense foods that provide essential minerals, vitamins, and healthy fats.

One simple strategy is to build each meal around the core components your body needs: proteins, healthy fats, and plenty of vegetables. These foods will provide the building blocks for long-term health, help regulate your blood pressure and keep you feeling satisfied.

Here's how you can approach meal planning with balance in mind:

- **Start with Protein**: Quality animal proteins like eggs, grass-fed beef, poultry, and fatty fish provide not only protein but also important vitamins and minerals like vitamin A, D, and omega-3 fatty acids. Include a palm-sized portion of protein in each meal to support muscle health, hormone production, and metabolism.
- **Add Healthy Fats**: Include a source of healthy fats in each meal, whether from olive oil, butter, avocados, or fatty fish. These fats will help you absorb fat-soluble vitamins (A, D, E, K) and keep you full longer, reducing the urge to snack on less healthy options.
- **Fill Your Plate with Vegetables**: Vegetables are essential for their fiber, vitamins, and mineral content. Leafy greens like spinach, kale, and Swiss

chard are rich in magnesium, potassium, and calcium, which are vital for controlling blood pressure. Aim to fill at least half your plate with a variety of colorful veggies. While raw vegetables offer certain nutrients in their most natural form, cooking vegetables can also enhance their benefits. Cooking can break down tough cell walls, making some nutrients more bioavailable. For example, cooking tomatoes increases the bioavailability of lycopene, a powerful antioxidant. Similarly, cooking leafy greens like spinach can enhance the absorption of calcium and iron. Cooking also aids digestion and supports gut health by making vegetables easier to break down, reducing potential digestive discomfort from raw veggies. By balancing raw and cooked vegetables in your meals, you can maximize nutrient absorption and support your overall health while keeping your diet varied and enjoyable.

- **Include Plenty of Fruits**: While fruits can provide necessary vitamins and fiber. Focus on those that are higher in nutrients, such as berries. Berries, such as blueberries, strawberries, and raspberries, are rich in antioxidants and have been shown to support cardiovascular health.

- **Choose Nutritious, Easily Digestible Carbohydrates**: Incorporating gluten-free carbohydrates like potatoes, rice, corn, and gluten-free pasta or breads provides essential nutrients such as magnesium, potassium, and fiber. These foods are not only filling but also easier on digestion, making them excellent options for supporting healthy blood pressure. Potatoes, in particular, are rich in potassium, while rice and corn offer energy-dense, gluten-free alternatives that help maintain a balanced diet without compromising gut health.

How to Plan Meals Around Essential Minerals and Vitamins

Balancing your meals with essential minerals and vitamins is crucial for long-term blood pressure control. Here's a quick guide on how to ensure your meals are packed with the nutrients you need:

- **Potassium**: Incorporate potassium-rich foods like avocados, sweet potatoes, bananas, and leafy greens into your meals. Potassium helps counterbalance sodium and supports heart health.
- **Magnesium**: Add magnesium-dense foods like almonds, spinach, quinoa, and dark chocolate to your diet.

Magnesium is essential for relaxing blood vessels and promoting healthy blood pressure.

- **Calcium**: While dairy products like yogurt and cheese are great sources of calcium, you can also get calcium from non-dairy sources like leafy greens (kale, collard greens), tofu, and fortified plant-based milk.
- **Fat-Soluble Vitamins**: Get your fat-soluble vitamins (A, D, E, K) from sources like fatty fish (for vitamin D), liver and eggs (for vitamin A), nuts and seeds (for vitamin E), and fermented foods like natto (for vitamin K2). Pair these with healthy fats for maximum absorption.

By incorporating these key nutrients into your meals, you'll create a powerful, balanced diet that supports your cardiovascular system and helps regulate blood pressure.

Recipes and Tips for Incorporating Leafy Greens, Fruits, Quality Animal Products, and Healthy Fats

To make these changes easier, here are a few practical recipes and tips that can seamlessly fit into your daily routine:

- **Breakfast**:
    - **Spinach and Mushroom Omelet**: Start your day with an omelet packed with spinach and mushrooms, cooked in butter or olive oil. Pair with a side of avocado for potassium and healthy fats.
    - **Overnight Oats with Berries**: Soak oats in almond milk overnight and top with chia seeds and blueberries. This provides a dose of magnesium, potassium, and antioxidants, keeping you full and energized.

- **Lunch**:
    - **Kale and Quinoa Salad**: Toss kale, cooked quinoa, sliced avocado, and grilled chicken together with a drizzle of olive oil and lemon juice. This meal provides essential minerals, healthy fats, and protein.
    - **Tuna Salad with Leafy Greens**: Mix canned tuna with olive oil, lemon, and a bit of mustard, then serve over a bed of mixed greens. Top with sunflower seeds for added vitamin E and magnesium.
- **Dinner**:
    - **Salmon with Roasted Vegetables**: Roast a fillet of wild-caught salmon with olive oil, garlic, and lemon. Serve with roasted Brussels sprouts and sweet potatoes for a nutrient-dense, satisfying meal rich in omega-3s, potassium, and magnesium.

- Beef Stir-Fry with Broccoli: Stir-fry strips of grass-fed beef with broccoli and bell peppers in coconut oil and serve over brown rice. This meal is full of protein, vitamins A and K, and heart-healthy fats.

By focusing on whole, nutrient-rich ingredients and preparing meals that include a balance of protein, fats, and vegetables, you can create sustainable eating habits that support blood pressure control.

Maintaining Long-Term Health with Simple Lifestyle Changes

Sustainable eating is about more than just food choices—it's about incorporating simple lifestyle changes that make it easier to maintain healthy habits over the long term. Here are a few tips to help you stay on track without feeling deprived:

1. **Meal Prep**: Take time each week to plan and prep your meals. Cook a batch of grains, roast vegetables, and pre-portion snacks like nuts or fruits to make healthy eating easy during busy days.
2. **Moderate Salt, Don't Eliminate It**: Use natural sea salt or Himalayan salt to season your meals. Salt in moderation, combined with potassium-rich foods, helps maintain a healthy sodium-potassium balance.
3. **Listen to Your Body**: Pay attention to hunger and fullness cues and focus on eating nourishing meals that leave you feeling satisfied. Avoid the trap of restrictive dieting, which can lead to frustration and unhealthy habits.
4. **Incorporate Physical Activity**: Regular exercise helps manage blood pressure, reduce stress, and improve overall heart health. Find activities you enjoy—whether it's walking,

swimming, or yoga—and make them a regular part of your routine.

<u>Reader Takeaway: Build a Balanced, Enjoyable Diet for Long-Term Health</u>

Sustainable eating isn't about strict rules or deprivation. It's about building a balanced, nutrient-rich diet that you can enjoy for the long term. By incorporating essential minerals, vitamins, and healthy fats into your meals, you can support cardiovascular health and maintain healthy blood pressure without feeling restricted.

The power to control your health is in your hands—and it starts with the simple, sustainable choices you make every day. Embrace whole foods, listen to your body, and allow these changes to become second nature as you work toward long-term wellness and balanced blood pressure.

Glossary

1. Aldosterone: A hormone that helps control blood pressure by regulating sodium and potassium levels in your body. Think of it as the body's way of balancing salts and water to keep your blood pressure steady.

2. Bioavailability: This refers to how well your body can absorb and use a nutrient. For example, cooking some vegetables can increase the bioavailability of certain vitamins, making it easier for your body to use them.

3. Catecholamines: These are hormones (like adrenaline) that are released during stress, which can raise your heart rate and

blood pressure. It's your body's "fight or flight" response kicking in.

4. Calcification: This happens when calcium builds up in soft tissues, like your arteries, making them stiff and hard. This is not a good thing because it can lead to heart problems by restricting blood flow.

5. Endotoxins: Toxic substances produced by certain bacteria in your gut. These can cause inflammation in your body and may negatively affect your heart health.

6. Electrolyte Balance: The balance of minerals like sodium, potassium, calcium, and magnesium in your body. These minerals control many important functions,

including keeping your heart and muscles working properly.

7. Fat-Soluble Vitamins (A, D, E, K): These are vitamins that dissolve in fat, not water, and are stored in your body's fatty tissues. You need to eat them with fats so your body can absorb and use them.

8. Hypertension: Another word for high blood pressure. It means that the force of blood pushing against the walls of your arteries is too high, which can lead to heart disease or stroke over time.

9. LDL/HDL Cholesterol: LDL is known as "bad" cholesterol because it can build up in your arteries, while HDL is "good"

cholesterol because it helps remove LDL from your bloodstream.

10. Magnesium: An essential mineral that helps relax blood vessels and muscles. It plays a major role in keeping your blood pressure in check and your heart healthy.

11. Mineralocorticoid Receptors: These are parts of your cells that respond to certain hormones (like aldosterone). They help control water and salt balance in your body, which affects blood pressure.

12. Nongenomic Effects: These are rapid actions that hormones can have on cells without changing your genes. It's like a fast-track response in your body that doesn't require any changes to your DNA.

13. Omega-3 Fatty Acids: Healthy fats found in fish and some plants that help lower inflammation and protect your heart by supporting good blood pressure and healthy cholesterol levels.

14. Parathyroid Function: The parathyroid glands control how much calcium is in your blood. If they are overactive, they can lead to calcium imbalances, which can affect your heart and bones.

15. Polyunsaturated Fatty Acids (PUFAs): Fats found in many vegetable oils. They are often considered healthy in small amounts but can cause problems when over-consumed, especially when used in processed foods.

16. Renin-Angiotensin System: A hormone system that helps regulate blood pressure and fluid balance in your body. When activated, it can cause blood vessels to tighten, raising your blood pressure.

17. Sodium-Potassium Pump (Na+-K+-ATPase): A process that keeps sodium and potassium balanced inside your cells. This pump is essential for maintaining proper heart function and keeping your blood pressure stable.

18. Trans Fats: Artificial fats found in processed foods that are harmful to your heart. They can increase bad cholesterol (LDL) and lower good cholesterol (HDL), leading to heart disease and hypertension.

19. Urinary Sodium Excretion: The amount of sodium (salt) your body gets rid of through urine. High sodium excretion can indicate you are consuming too much salt, which may raise your blood pressure.

Bibliography

I've tried to keep this book as simple and practical as possible, avoiding medical jargon and statistical overload so you can focus on the actionable steps to better manage your blood pressure. But for those of you with an affinity for scientific details and a desire to explore the research behind these ideas, I've provided the key studies and concepts here.

If you'd like to expand on any of the ideas discussed throughout the book, the following End Notes will guide you to the scientific backing behind each concept.

1. Graudal, N. A., Galløe, A. M., & Garred, P. (1998).

Effects of sodium restriction on blood pressure, renin, aldosterone, catecholamines, cholesterol, and triglyceride: A meta-analysis. JAMA, 279(17), 1383-1391.

   - This study provides essential insight into how sodium restriction impacts various cardiovascular and metabolic markers, helping us question conventional low-sodium advice.

2. Horton, R., & Biglieri, E. G. (1962).

   Effect of aldosterone on the metabolism of magnesium. The Journal of Clinical Endocrinology & Metabolism, 22(12), 1187-1192.

   - Here, the role of aldosterone and magnesium balance is examined, which is crucial for understanding hypertension regulation via mineral balance.

3. Mihailidou, A. S., & Funder, J. W. (2005).

Nongenomic effects of mineralocorticoid receptor activation in the cardiovascular system. Steroids, 70(5-7), 347-351.

- This research explores how mineralocorticoid receptors influence the cardiovascular system, a key point when discussing hypertension's deeper metabolic causes.

4. Cohen, H. W., Hailpern, S. M., Fang, J., & Alderman, M. H. (2006).

Sodium intake and mortality in the NHANES II follow-up study. The American Journal of Medicine, 119(3), 275.e7-275.e14.

- This study examines the complex relationship between sodium intake and mortality, challenging the one-size-fits-all approach to sodium and hypertension.

5. Stolarz-Skrzypek, K., Kuznetsova, T., Thijs, L., Tikhonoff, V., Seidlerová, J., Richart, T., Jin, Y., Olszanecka, A., Malyutina, S., Casiglia, E., Filipovský, J., Kawecka-Jaszcz, K., Nikitin, Y., & Staessen, J. A. (2011).

 Fatal and nonfatal outcomes, incidence of hypertension, and blood pressure changes in relation to urinary sodium excretion. JAMA, 305(17), 1777-1785.

   - This research ties sodium excretion directly to blood pressure outcomes, expanding the discussion on sodium balance rather than strict reduction.

6. O'Donnell, M. J., Yusuf, S., Mente, A., Gao, P., Mann, J. F., Teo, K., McQueen, M., Sleight, P., Sharma, A. M., Dans, A., Probstfield, J., & Schmieder, R. E. (2011).

Urinary sodium and potassium excretion and risk of cardiovascular events. JAMA, 306(20), 2229-2238.

- A key study linking sodium and potassium excretion with cardiovascular risks, emphasizing the importance of mineral balance in hypertension management.

7. Haddy, F. J. (1982).

Potassium effects on contraction in arterial smooth muscle mediated by Na+-K+-ATPase. Journal of Cardiovascular Pharmacology, 4(Suppl 1), S134-S143.

- This study explains how potassium plays a critical role in smooth muscle contraction, which is directly linked to blood pressure regulation.

8. Krishna, G. G. (1990).

Effect of potassium intake on blood pressure. Journal of the American Society of Nephrology: JASN, 1(1), 43-52.

- Krishna's research on potassium's effects on blood pressure underpins much of our discussion about balancing sodium with potassium in the diet.

9. McCarron, D. A., Pingree, P. A., Rubin, R. J., Gaucher, S. M., Molitch, M., & Krutzik, S. (1980).

Enhanced parathyroid function in essential hypertension: A homeostatic response to a urinary calcium leak. Hypertension, 2(2), 162-168.

- This study provides an essential understanding of calcium's role in hypertension, especially in cases linked to abnormal calcium metabolism.

10. McCarron, D. A., Morris, C. D., Bukoski, R., & Stanton, J. L. (1987).

The calcium paradox of essential hypertension. The American Journal of Medicine, 82(1B), 27-33.

- Further expanding on the role of calcium, this study introduces the "calcium paradox" and its impact on hypertension, reinforcing the importance of balanced nutrient intake.

11. Jane AH Masoli, Joao Delgado, Luke Pilling, David Strain, David Melzer (2020).

Blood pressure in frail older adults: associations with cardiovascular outcomes and all-cause mortality. Age and Ageing, 2020; 49: 807–813

- The study concludes that lowering systolic blood pressure to below 130 mmHg in frail older adults, particularly those over 75, may increase mortality, with the lowest all-cause mortality observed in individuals maintaining systolic pressures between 140-160 mmHg.

www.ingramcontent.com/pod-product-compliance
Lightning Source LLC
Chambersburg PA
CBHW050813250726

48653CB00006B/2207